Don't Be Social Tofu

...and hundreds of other smart weight loss tactics for silencing the devil on your shoulder

Jill Brook, M.A.

IBSN 978-0-9830941-3-5

Published by YAMBE Press
at
www.dietforhealth.com

This book is intended solely as a general reference and
should not be used as a substitute for medical advice or
treatment. Some supplements, fruits and teas may
interact with certain medications, so be sure to check
with your doctor first before making any changes to
your diet. Also, for your safety it is strongly
recommended that you get your doctor's approval
before beginning any new exercise activities.

Book design and cover by Melissa Darnell

Table of Contents

Foreword

Hello, it's Jill here, and I'm writing this to end the misery for every educated eater out there feeling guilty about their imperfect habits and weight. I want to make you think differently about eating, exercise and weight loss so you can lose the guilt and find your solution. My experience with 5,000 clients, who have lost over 100,000 pounds, proves that a simple shift in focus can make all the difference.

I know you're already working hard to eat right and lose weight. The strategies in this book will help you work smarter, so that the valuable time, energy and willpower you invest will pay off with more permanent success.

Introduction

It's a bloodbath out there: With each passing year we're trying harder to lose weight, yet we're still gaining over 2 pounds per year, on average. Yikes! Are we really that pathetic? Of course not. What's pathetic is our approach to weight loss. It's time to accept that the conventional weight loss approach is fatally flawed.

We're doing it wrong.

We're suffering needlessly: We're wasting time, money, and willpower, and still feeling deprived and experiencing unnecessary guilt. This whole fiasco is hurting our mental health as much as our physical health, and it breaks my heart to see so many smart, ambitious, high-achieving people feeling terrible about themselves over their repeated failures. The problem isn't us; it's our approach.

You've probably seen this quote:

"Grant me the courage to change what I can, the serenity to accept what I can't, and the wisdom to know the difference."

This quote perfectly explains America's weight failure: We're tirelessly working to change what we *can't*. That leaves us exhausted and frustrated in a futile fight. In addition, we're failing to focus our energies on the many factors we *can* change, and missing out on the success it would bring.

I'm writing this book to help you re-direct your energy into the things that you can control, which will help bring you long-term success. I also hope to free you of the burden of trying to control what you can't.

5,000 clients have taught me that our willpower doesn't have as much control over our behavior as we'd like to believe; and our biological instincts have more.

How many times do you have to "give in" to your hunger, cravings, sweet tooth, etc. before you conclude that you can not—I repeat, CAN NOT—win that battle? We've all lost it a thousand times and yet we keep blaming ourselves, insisting that if we work hard enough, we can win this fight. I'm here to tell you to lose the guilt because it's not winnable. It's like trying to use willpower to stifle an imminent sneeze that's already in your lungs; once your sneezing response is triggered, willpower alone can't change it.

Did you get that? This is important. In my experience with helping thousands of people fight biological instincts, like cravings, hunger, a sweet tooth, etc., I find that:

These biological instincts, once set in motion, are awfully hard to change. You'll waste a lot of willpower trying.

So, what *can* we change? Lots of things! It turns out that there are many factors—within our control—that determine whether our hunger, cravings, sweet tooth, and other fat-loving instincts get triggered in the first place. It's like stopping that same sneeze by getting an air purifier. We can stop this uncontrollable biological response from ever getting started.

With this smarter approach to managing your weight, your effort doesn't go into *fighting* hunger, cravings, sweet tooth, and all the other biology that works against you. Instead, your effort goes into preventing the fight in the first place. The key is this:

Rather than focusing on just *eating right*, you focus on *making your body want to*.

With this approach, your efforts buy you more long-term success and less long-term struggle. You've got a goal you can achieve within a month or two, instead of a lifelong battle. You employ cooperation and finesse instead of brute force. It's still a lot of work. But by training your body to want to eat right and exercise, the work is finite. After the training is done, you're just doing what you like to do and eating how you like to eat.

5,000 clients have taught me that this is the Smarter Way.

CHAPTER 1:
Choose Finesse Over Force

"If you want to be incrementally better: Be competitive. If you want to be exponentially better: Be cooperative." -Unknown

Knowing how to lose weight isn't usually enough, no matter how brilliant and ambitious you might be. *Knowing* is simple: eat less and move more. Different experts may give slightly different opinions on the details, but we all know the true path to weight loss: eat less junky stuff, drink less fun stuff, eat more veggies and exercise more. The problem is that knowing doesn't help much with the hard part of weight loss: **doing it.**

Knowing how to lose weight mostly helps with...

...Producing guilt!

In most areas of life, once you know how and why to do something important, you will do it. Brushing your teeth, wearing a seatbelt, changing your oil, finishing projects at work on time are all examples of where most people find it relatively easy to practice what they know they *should*. How come eating and exercise are so different?

Nature.

It's because, in weight loss, the actions you must take—eating fewer calories and expending more—go against many of your body's natural instincts. Mother Nature has devised many tricks to make you as plump as possible: she gave you taste buds that love junk food, an appetite that doesn't quit, irresistible cravings, a metabolism that slows down any chance it gets, and willpower that is no match for today's environment that practically shovels food down your throat. It's as if Mother Nature herself put the devil on your shoulder, bidding you to falter.

What a raw deal! Why would nature design a system so stacked against our weight loss success?!

Survival.

Unfortunately, we're up against a most powerful force driving our instincts. The weight loss saboteur is in our very bodies: our stomachs, taste buds, hormones, muscles and even in parts of our brains.

Our biology is designed to help us gain weight. Even when we have high cholesterol, triglycerides or aching joints telling us we should lose weight.

Our biology always works toward weight gain.

Here's why: our biology has spent millions of years trying to survive in an environment where food was scarce, life was harsh, and exercise was a daily necessity. Some anthropologists have estimated that early man walked an average of 12 miles per day carrying 25 pounds, and then had to do *more* exercise to chop, cook and complete other chores of living. Researchers have also estimated that the average well-fed human ate about 1500 calories per day.

Did you get that? That's 1,500 calories on a good day, with many hours of strenuous exercise. Are you hungry just thinking about it?   Those were the conditions our biology dealt with, until a few hundred years ago, when humans got much better at making food available. Because a few hundred years is not enough time for our biology to change, we've still got instincts geared for the ever-present threat of starvation.

In that "starved" environment, humans never had a reason to resist food. If an early human had a chance to eat 500 extra calories, with little effort, that was a potentially life-saving gift. Early humans also had no reason to exercise for any reason other than survival. Anybody doing "caveman aerobics" was wasting valuable energy, increasing their chances for starvation. I imagine that Jane Fonda, Jennifer Aniston, and many more of today's top models would have been goners for sure, had they lived in an earlier time!

Imagine an early human running for days to chase down a buffalo, risking his life to kill it, dragging it back to his family and then knowing he's got to do it all over again the next time he wants to eat. Or, if he wanted a single ounce of pumpkin seeds (under 200 calories), he'd need to find, cut open and clean an entire messy, slimy pumpkin (without nice kitchen knives!) and dry out the seeds for weeks. Every Halloween, when I do this ritual, I am reminded of what a measly food pay-off our ancestors got for their hard work.

Anyway, you get the idea. In an environment where food is scarce and you risk your life to get more, overeating is a rare and valuable opportunity. Any free calorie or nutrient is a gift!

It makes sense that willpower was never intended to help us avoid eating or get us to the gym—Nature rewarded the lazy overeaters and killed off the people who exercised too much or ate too little.

So thank your ancestors for being lazy overeaters every (rare) chance they got...because you probably wouldn't be here otherwise!

In other words, the fat-loving biology you hate is the same biology that got you here today. So instead of feeling guilty about your ability to love junk food, overeat, or under-move, just recognize that our problem these days is *that our environment changed, but our biology didn't.*

It is biologically natural to want to overeat and load up on sugar, fat, salt and processed food. It's natural to eat when stressed, bored or any time some food is available. It's natural to tend to finish off the leftovers rather than throw them away. It's natural to eat when you aren't hungry, and it's natural to prefer junk food over vegetables. It's natural to want to lie on the sofa rather than exercise. It's natural to socialize with your personal trainer to try to delay that next set of squats. It's natural to gorge yourself.

What isn't natural is an environment that allows you to do these things.

As long as you try to fight your biology, you are doomed to ultimately fail. Willpower can be strong, but biology is always stronger. Biology is at work every minute of the day, week and year, and even the strongest willpower can't match that. Those few moments, when willpower takes a break, will be enough for your fat-loving instincts to consume enough pizza, crackers or name-your-vice to put on some weight. You know this already. Those 5 minutes every Friday afternoon (or whenever you break down), when you have a treat (that can snowball into a double-treat or worse), prove it time and again.

Your biology is very powerful. Willpower is no match for it. Biology, in the long run, will always win.

But there is a solution!

Instead of fighting biological instincts—and losing—we can avoid the fight altogether. If we use finesse instead of force, if we get our instincts working *for* us instead of *against* us, we have a much better chance of success. This book will teach you how to do just that. It will show you how to:

- reduce the strength and frequency of cravings

- get your taste buds to quit crying out for sweet, salty or rich foods

- get your stomach to feel satisfied on fewer calories and less quantity

- keep your metabolism going strong

- make exercise truly enjoyable

- strengthen your willpower, and

- manage your environments to be a better influence

Fortunately, researchers have been studying how to best accomplish these things. Their studies have led to the discovery of many effective tricks and strategies, which are the smart ways to lose weight permanently.

When you've trained your instincts to *want* to eat right, *prefer* to eat less, and *enjoy* vigorous exercise, you make it much easier to reach your goal weight and *stay* there. I'm convinced that this is the only way to lose weight, because the alternative requires you to continually do what you'd rather not. *That's no way to live!*

The following chapters share my best advice for training your biological instincts to work for you, rather than against you. My positive experience with 5,000 clients has taught me that focusing your willpower and efforts on these strategies, rather than just fighting to make it through another day of dieting, is the smarter way.

CHAPTER 2:
Calm Your Cravings

Even when you manage to resist a craving, it wears you down. It weakens your willpower, makes you feel deprived and eventually makes you feel like giving up. Let's get rid of these nasty buggers!

The first step to managing cravings is to understand them. Like an enemy to be defeated, it helps to know their motives and methods, and to have a healthy appreciation for their strength and resourcefulness.

Many cravings are probably caused by your body's wisdom. For example, when you are dehydrated you may crave salt, which makes you thirsty and helps you retain needed water. That's not a design flaw—that's smart biology. When you have low blood-sugar, you crave calories that will raise it quickly—again, smart biology. When your brain senses stress, pain or depression, you crave "comfort foods" that will make your brain release chemicals that calm and cheer you. What a sophisticated body!

The only problem is that our cravings tend to overreact and to focus only on our immediate needs. They call out for more salt, sugar or comfort food than we really need and ignore the fact that we want to stay lean in the long-run.

That's smart biology in the world of the past, where life expectancy was short and any given instance of low blood sugar or salt deficiency could mean death. Survival was much more a matter of surviving this day or hour, and much less surviving to old age with clean arteries. In the world of the past, it could take days to find food that would raise your blood sugar or provide necessary salt. And you'd be getting weaker with each passing hour, making it all the harder to solve your problem.

You may be asking, "So why don't I crave vegetables? I need those to be healthy!" And you'd be correct that they are essential for optimal health. The likely reasons we don't crave them is that the nutrients provided in vegetables are not the kind that determined one's immediate survival. The minerals, antioxidants, phytonutrients, and fiber in veggies make you age well, but they don't determine whether you can outrun a tiger today or walk 20 miles to find food. Plus, these plant-based nutrients were often the easiest to come by in earlier times, so they were rarely the limiting factor to one's health. Early people probably ran out of carbs, calories, protein and salt before they suffered from lack of veggies, so Nature never needed to worry about the latter. Nature developed cravings as alarm bells to tell you what it needs *right now*.

Of course, cravings aren't as smart as we'd like them to be. They don't know that we've got plenty of calories stored on our hips. All they know is that when blood sugar drops, they set off the alarms. It's a system that worked great throughout most of prehistory; it just doesn't work great now.

When you think of cravings in these terms, you almost have to admire them. And then you have to get to work minimizing them!

Here are my best tips for preventing, reducing and managing cravings:

Prevent the needs and imbalances that create most cravings in the first place.

This may seem obvious, but most people get sloppy and don't realize the consequences. If you stay well-hydrated, you'll crave less salt. If you keep your blood sugar up, you'll prevent sweet cravings. If you avoid sleep-deprivation, exhaustion, extreme stress, pain and injury, your brain won't call out for comfort foods. With cravings, an ounce of prevention might just be worth a pound of soon-to-be-regretted Oreos.

It seems odd that us well-fed Americans could be lacking necessary nutrients, but actually we are notorious for being "overfed, but undernourished." But you can fix that!

- Be aware of habits that may dehydrate you, like drinking alcohol, coffee, tea, soda or sweating or taking diuretics. Keep in mind that many "diet teas" or other products are diuretic—that's how they get you to lose some quick weight. Drink extra water to replace lost fluids, and also eat foods full of water and electrolytes, like veggies and fresh fruits.

- Don't let your blood sugar get low. Eat a snack every few hours to keep it up. Some people need to eat even more often. Get to know your body and then eat as often as you need to. If you have very finicky blood sugar, get a nutritionist to help you get it under control.

- Eat enough protein each day. If you are an American, you are probably eating plenty, if not *too* much, but it's worth checking. Aim for a daily intake of about .8g protein per kilogram (2.2lbs) of *healthy* body weight.

- Eat so many varied nutritious foods that your body will have regular access to every nutrient it could possibly need. Vitamin supplements are not the same. Nutrients from real foods are much better.

- Eat enough calcium from green veggies, dairy, tofu or quality supplements, as low blood levels of calcium have been linked to cravings for fatty foods. The theory is that your body craves rich foods like ice cream, cheese, or cream because they contain the calcium your body needs.

- Let your body have adequate rest and relaxation whenever possible, to avoid stress-cravings.

- Avoid pain when possible. Even if you hate taking pain relievers, it might be sometimes worth it if the alternative is constant cravings.

You can prevent need-based cravings if you take good care of your body and never let any dire needs arise in the first place.

This means it's not selfish to take excellent care of yourself! Spending time, energy and money on your nutrition, relaxation and comfort is not decadent; it's smarter weight loss.

Understand—and then avoid—self-medication.

It is well-known that eating tasty food—especially carbohydrates—makes your brain release chemicals like serotonin that make you feel happy and/or calm. Even if *you* don't consciously know this, your brain and taste buds sure do.

These smart little guys crave carbohydrates when they want to boost your mood and/or put you at ease. How smart of them! The only problem is that they don't realize they are causing you more unhappiness and stress in the long run by keeping you from losing weight. Here's how to prevent these cravings:

Boost serotonin through other, weight-friendly means. Here are some:

- laughter

- healthy touch (massage, cuddling, hugs, consensual sex)

- meditation, prayer, positive visualization

- exercise

- listening to pleasant music

- interaction with pleasant people and pets

- sunshine

- calming hobbies—anything you enjoy

- adequate intake of b-vitamins, magnesium, calcium (i.e., keep eating healthy)

The only problem: most of these things don't boost your mood as quickly as your favorite junky food does. So plan ahead and have a few of these activities planned every week so that your serotonin never gets too low in the first place.

With many clients, I have seen their cravings melt away when they schedule a weekly massage, bubble bath, yoga class, etc. Friday night is a perfect time for this regular activity, because it helps erase the stress of the week and puts you in a strong anti-craving position for the weekend. If you're married, do it with your spouse and see how great it feels to decompress together and start the weekend out right.

Once a craving strikes, don't overcompensate...despite your pleading brain.

If you are diabetic, follow your doctor's instructions for low blood sugar. This tip is only for non-diabetics.

When your blood sugar gets a little low, it can feel like you need a thousand calories to feel good again. This translates into a strong craving because your brain, which relies on blood sugar as its only source of fuel, is at risk for running out of energy. This is why your mood, memory, and concentration all suffer, as it shuts down some nonessential functions. Your brain then rings an alarm in the form of a craving too strong to ignore.

It says (to me, anyway) "let's eat a bathtub full of cereal, then a loaf of bread, then last night's leftover lasagna, then we'll decide on dessert!"

Don't listen—your brain is overreacting. Despite the fact that you crave a boatload of calories, you don't need them. In fact, your blood stream can only hold about 40-60 calories at a time anyway! Your brain can be back-in-business with a single slice of toast.

Here's what to do: eat a high-glycemic (quick-digesting) 40-100 calories of carbohydrates—like a couple of rice cakes, a handful of grapes or slice of bread. That should get you feeling good again in a few minutes. Just make sure to eat a healthy snack soon, because the 40-100 calories won't hold you for long.

If you are prone to low blood sugar, make sure to eat more frequent small snacks and consider leaving some "emergency" snacks in your desk, glove compartment, brief case and purse. (If this happens during exercise, that's a different situation and you need lots more calories.)

Go to bed

Here's a research note that may ring true for you: most cravings happen after dark. For a yet unknown reason, after sundown your craving demons come out! What to do? Go to bed as early as possible and don't spend Christmas in Alaska!

Salt smarts

While not proven, many Nutritionists believe that a craving for salt is often your body's way of letting you know it's dehydrated. Eating salt helps hydrate you because it is an electrolyte and also makes you thirsty.

Next time you crave salt, go ahead and have some, but choose *foods that are both rich in salt and healthy*, not chips and munchy snacks. Top choices are:

- vegetable soup

- salted steamed veggies

- pickles

- hearts of palm

- artichoke hearts

- nonfat cottage cheese

- low-fat string cheese

- a salad with salsa, salt or low-cal salty dressing (almost all dressings are salty)

- tuna

In addition to being lower in calories, these foods also contain minerals and electrolytes that help keep you hydrated.

Don't play taste bud ping pong.

Any extreme flavor will make you crave the opposite flavor. This explains a lot, right? This is why pastries are so tempting when you drink coffee and why you may crave movie popcorn with your diet soda. Do you always crave sweets after eating (salt-laden) Chinese food? Many people do.

Flavors and their opposites:

Salty and sweet

- French fries and a shake

- diet soda and movie popcorn

- peanut butter and jelly

- pizza sauce and cheese

Bitter and sweet

- coffee and donut

- chocolate (both flavors combined)

- frappucino

Prevent these ping-pong cravings by avoiding that first over-flavored food that gets you started. Priority one is to stop drinking sweet beverages, even those that are calorie-free, if they make you crave salty foods later on. Look out for other extreme flavors in your diet, some of which may seem so harmless! For example, the deli turkey meat or the soy sauce on your veggies can't be that bad, right? Right...unless they catapult you to the next craving for the opposite flavor. Try using just enough salt, sweet or bitter flavor to satisfy your taste buds and *no extra*.

Many people plagued by cravings are simply sensitive to taste bud ping pong. I've had clients who got rid of cravings simply by switching to a natural, less-sweet toothpaste. Also, many people who think they only crave salt (and not sweets) don't realize that their diet drinks—which they don't even notice as sweet—are causing their problems.

Pay attention and see if you need to start your day with blander food and drink. It may make a huge difference all day long by preventing the ping pong game from even starting.

Avoid the Trifecta.

New research is suggesting that there is a flavor combination that can hold your brain hostage until you've eaten as much as you can stuff in your stretched-out stomach. This nasty combo apparently over-stimulates our brains and makes us nearly obsessed, unable to think about much else. It's the combination of salt, fat and carbohydrate. Examples are:

- pizza

- donuts (yes, they have salt)

- frosting (ditto on the salt)

- hamburgers, fries and a coke

- ice cream (check out the sodium)

- most restaurant meals, processed foods, and everything that is crazy-delicious

Researchers have found that when a food with this combination is present, the pleasure center in our brain goes wild and secretes dopamine, a neurotransmitter that focuses attention on the tasty treat... which explains why certain foods "call out" to you if they are anywhere within your grasp.

What can you do? Well, until researchers find the cure, the best thing is to keep these irresistible foods out of your reach. Ban them. Shun them. Think of them like crack cocaine. I wish there was a better solution, but for now it's our only hope.

Craving-Prevention To-Do List

- Take stock of your diet and see if you are missing any food groups or nutrients. A qualified Nutritionist or online nutrition program can help you identify any gaps.

- Get to the grocery store and stock up on super-nutritious foods. Make sure to include some calcium-rich foods and the healthy salty foods mentioned in this chapter, if you sometimes crave salt.

- Make (and protect!) time in your upcoming schedule for weekly relaxation, pampering and sleep.

- Make a list of comforting things you can do next time you need to self-medicate without food.

- Put some "emergency snacks" in your office, car, purse or other places you might find yourself with low blood sugar.

Craving Conclusions

These tips involve using your effort and willpower to *prevent* the conditions that cause cravings, rather than battle them once they've grown fierce. This is the smarter way, because it's a tough battle, and your willpower will often lose.

CHAPTER 3:
Tame Your Taste Buds

Don't be at the mercy of insatiable taste buds! Understand them and then train them to be great little weight loss helpers.

Your taste buds undermine your weight loss efforts for one reason: survival.

Until recently, when safe, clean, and fresh food became *over*abundant, the taste buds helped to make sure you sought out enough energy and nutrients to live on without eating anything poisonous or rotten. Remember, your ancestors were finding food wherever they could—it wasn't always clean, fresh and appealing. You can bet that when times were tough, people were eating foods that are pretty sketchy by our standards. Slightly moldy nuts, meat with a few insects on it, or bruised overripe apples probably looked delicious to people who hadn't eaten in a few days!

Kooky Factoid:

You've probably heard of Civil War re-enactors who meet to relive the battles and everyday life of that time period, 1861-1864. While reading about them, I was struck by a funny factoid: in an effort to be more realistic, the more serious participants will not allow themselves to bring any modern foods. Not only can't they bring sandwiches or trail mix, but they can't even bring nice fruit. To be historically accurate, they must bring only mealy, bruised, over- or under-ripe apples, since that was the norm back then. Under-ripe corn was another staple, which is interesting because it's barely digestible and causes diarrhea. But that was often their only choice back then...and that wasn't so long ago. That sure makes me appreciate my shiny, fresh apples!

Anyway, your taste buds were designed to protect you by guiding you to the safe and energy-dense foods.

The different basic tastes are thought to correspond to different important substances or properties that humans needed to either consume or avoid:

Salty taste is pleasant because it indicates the presence of sodium, which is essential for mammals to stay hydrated. Even though we get too much of it

---

nowadays, earlier humans were constantly in danger of getting too little. In fact, it is said that early Roman soldiers were sometimes paid for their work with salt instead of money—that's where the word *salary* comes from.

So, once again, our biology is brilliant; that is, for a low-salt environment that doesn't exist anymore. In today's super-salted environment, our taste buds tend to get us in trouble.

Sweet taste signals the presence of carbohydrates, which are your body's preferred energy source. For millions of years, when humans didn't know when they'd get a chance to eat again, it made sense to load up on carbs whenever possible.

In addition, it is widely believed that we are born with a sweet tooth to ensure that babies will drink their mother's milk. That certainly helps survival.

Also, consider what the sweetest available foods were to earlier human: fruit! Yes, boring old fruit, and not the super-sweet, big, domesticated kind we have today. Today's fruit has been carefully bred to taste great. Yesteryear's fruits contained even less carbohydrates and were not very caloric compared to today's fruits; much less compared to today's cookies, candies and Death by Chocolate Cake.

So your sweet-loving taste buds were helpful way-back-when, and couldn't get you into too much trouble. ...unlike today.

Umami, or savory, taste indicates the presence of the amino acid L-glutamate—i.e. protein. Americans today eat loads of animal protein by global and historical standards. We eat so much that early man would salivate with jealousy.

Early man probably couldn't get enough protein, especially because animals were not only hard to catch, but also smaller and skinnier than today's overfed, sedentary, farm-raised animals. Early animals were struggling for survival, just like everyone else, and rarely had an opportunity to eat enough, so they were scrawny and didn't have any nice fat marbling their flesh. So when you imagine cave men eating steaks over an open flame, remember they were very small, lean, tough steaks. With no salt or seasonings...bummer for them!

Early man also needed more protein than we do because he was exercising so much more and probably incurring more injuries (hey, who wouldn't fall or twist an ankle now and then, hunting and foraging all day with primitive tools, on uneven terrain, among predators, without hiking boots?)

If early man was walking or running an average of 12 miles per day, carrying 25 pounds, and then also doing all kinds of physical activity to survive, it's safe to say he had lots of sore muscles and frequent injuries. Eating adequate protein meant he had the building blocks necessary to heal his wounds and repair his tissues, whereas lack of protein meant that he was quickly becoming a damaged and easy-to-catch meal for some predator.

Females had extra protein needs for growing a healthy fetus and then breastfeeding her infants. This means women had an extra incentive to love the savory/umami taste that they could only get from protein.

In the end, the umami-loving humans had a valuable survival edge, so now we're left with taste buds that adore the stuff.

Incidentally, MSG has this taste. That's why we love it so much.

Sour taste is usually unpleasant because it can signal over-ripe fruit, rotten meat, and other spoiled foods, which can be dangerous to the body because of bacteria which grow in such conditions. Sour flavor can also indicate strong acidity, which can cause serious tissue damage.

Nowadays we don't taste many spoiled foods, thanks to refrigeration and preservatives. That has enabled us to acquire a liking for sour foods, like yogurt or sour candies. But historically, sour taste meant "Danger! Do not eat!"

Bitter taste is usually unpleasant (unless it becomes an "acquired taste", like beer or coffee) because it seems to be a warning that a substance may be toxic, poisonous or have drug-like affects. Nicotine, caffeine, pesticide, strychnine and many drugs have a bitter taste. Again, your taste buds are protecting you from eating something harmful.

Other tastes, such as that of "water" (yes, apparently it has a taste) or "calcium" are being discovered, and all of them seem to be your mouth's way of getting you to eat more of the important nutrients for survival. Nature never expected us to have too many nutrients and calories. She prepared us only for famine by making our taste buds scream with pleasure whenever they get salt, sugar, protein and energy (calories). No wonder junk food tastes so good!

Fortunately, there are some ways to calm down those taste buds and make them stop wanting so much junk. Here are my best ways to do it:

Understand habituation, also called adaptation.

When taste buds are repeatedly exposed to a strong flavor, they change and become temporarily less sensitive to that flavor. For example, this means that if you eat something very sweet for breakfast (like a sweet cereal) you may desensitize your taste buds to the point that your morning apple tastes bland. If you had eaten unsweetened cereal for breakfast, that same apple would taste much sweeter.

Learn to know when your taste buds have become desensitized, like after a rich meal or after that unintended pig-out. You'll know because foods that used to taste good now taste bland. At this time it's important not to add more sugar, fat, or salt! You could keep adding more in search of that good flavor, but your taste buds will just keep getting more desensitized. Instead, be patient and eat "clean" for the rest of the day. Yes, your food will taste bland, but that's the price you pay. By morning, your taste buds will be more sensitive again.

Grow virgin taste buds to get more flavor from your food.

A dentist once taught me this super-valuable factoid: taste buds are like hair; they live for a few weeks and then are replaced by fresh, new ones.

Use this to your advantage: any time your taste buds stop cooperating with your healthy diet (i.e., they ask for more sugar, fat, salt, etc.), you can trade them in for fresh new ones. It just takes a little patience.

If you invest a week or two in eating "clean", it gives your tongue time to grow new, virgin, extra-sensitive taste-buds. The old ones (which have been desensitized by intense salty, sweet, savory, etc. flavors) will find healthy food bland. But don't give in! Avoid over-flavored junk for 1-4 weeks—the lifespan of a taste-bud cell—and see how healthy foods become more flavorful again. Brown rice will taste nutty, carrots sweet, onions salty. In the end, you'll be more satisfied with healthy foods.

Use the 90% solution.

Almost all of the flavor of any food comes in the first few bites. After that, your taste buds adapt to the flavor and stop giving you much bang for your buck (or *flavor* for your *calorie*!). Whenever you are eating cookies, cake, chips or other junk, savor those first few bites—which contain all the flavor—and then fill up on something healthier.

Avoid taste bud ping pong.

When you eat foods with opposite tastes—think of salty French fries with sweet ketchup, bitter coffee with a sweet pastry—both foods taste better, which makes it harder to stop eating. In fact, studies show that the pleasure center of your brain gets over-stimulated, making it almost impossible to stop. Try to eat only one flavor at a time if you're at risk for overeating. Be especially careful at bars and restaurants, where this method is often used to get you to eat and drink more. Ever wonder why salty nuts and pretzels are free at bars?!

Exploit exercise effects.

Exercise makes flavors taste stronger. It also makes people enjoy watery foods (i.e. fruits and veggies) more. Use this to your advantage by eating fruit and veggies after working out. In fact, sweets and salty snacks should taste over-flavored after a workout and, if they don't, go back to the earlier tip about growing virgin taste buds.

Bore them into submission.

Some folks find that if they eat similar flavors all day (e.g. tomato omelet at breakfast, tomato soup at lunch, chicken with marinara sauce at dinner, etc.) they will eat less and be satisfied with less food. The lack of variety prevents your brain from getting over-stimulated by food and so it is easier to stop eating as soon as you are satisfied.

Eat healthiest when hungriest.

Your taste buds seem to become extra fond of whatever foods you eat when you are at your hungriest, regardless of whether it's junk food or health food. This is probably because you develop a positive association between that food and satisfying a great need. Use this to your advantage by making sure you have good choices available for those hungry times. For example, are you always starved when you get home from work? Then keep an "emergency salad" or other healthy choice in your fridge, ready to go the minute you walk in. Before you know it, you'll be loving salads more than ever!

Use natural toothpaste...

...instead of over-flavored, over-stimulating popular brands, which blitz your tongue and cause adaptation to sweet flavors. You don't want to start your day by desensitizing your taste buds, so brush your teeth with a small amount of naturally-flavored toothpaste, and do it after breakfast. This will allow any breakfast foods to be more flavorful.

Don't over-flavor breakfast.

For the same reason just mentioned, save the artificial sweeteners, salt and sugar for later in the day...if you must have them at all. This will keep your taste-buds more sensitive for a more satisfying day of eating "clean" foods.

Heat the sweet.

Any sweet food tastes sweeter when warm, and less sweet when cold. That's bad news for ice cream lovers because it means that you are consuming more sugar for less flavor. Switching to hot cocoa will allow you to cut down the sugar and keep the sweet taste. This goes for any food, so try adding less sugar to your pies, cookies or cakes (if you *must* eat them) and then heat them before eating.

Taste Bud To-Do List

- Buy natural toothpaste, like Tom's of Maine.

- Buy new breakfast foods if you need to find a new breakfast (or breakfast beverage) that is less sweet or salty. My suggestions: eggs, fresh fruit, Ezekiel toast, old fashioned oats, nonfat plain yogurt (sweeten it yourself with fruit or the smallest amount of sweetener that will satisfy).

- Buy a replacement for diet soda or other overly sweet foods and drinks. Try iced tea, diluted Crystal Light or, ideally, water.

- Start using the smallest possible amount of salt and sweetener to make your foods palatable. Better yet, go cold turkey and clean up your taste buds quickly.

Taste Bud Conclusions

Your weight loss efforts are well rewarded when you work to sensitize your taste-buds, to make healthy foods delicious and even preferable. Otherwise, without your taste-buds preferring to eat "clean", you'll forever have to rely on willpower to choose healthy foods that taste bland to you.

CHAPTER 4:
Appease Your Appetite

You can't go through life hungry! Luckily, you don't have to.

In Okinawa, where there are more centenarians than anywhere else, people stop eating when they are 80% full. How do they do that?!

For most of us in America today, food has never been scarce. We've never needed to eat as much food as possible to store excess energy as fat for the sake of surviving a day, a week, or longer without food. Let's be thankful for that.

Now imagine a time when your pantry wasn't full of non-perishables and there were no grocery stores. This time wasn't too long ago. There were a lot of reasons why you might not get to eat again for a day or week or longer. Some of the reasons were:

- drought

- flood

- winter

- insect infestation

- competition for food

- disease among the plants or animals you wanted to eat

- your food stores could be stolen

- you could be injured, sick or too tired to look for food

- A bad storm could keep you from hunting and gathering.

- A smarter and faster person could have hunted and gathered all the available food in the area.

That's a lot of very realistic possibilities! No wonder Mother Nature gave us expandable stomachs and the desire to fill them. No wonder she made it possible to store extra food energy in a light and highly-portable way: fat.

Fun Factoid:

One pound of body fat is the size of 4 sticks of butter and contains 3,500 calories. Fat is basically an extra fuel tank for your body, and it's wonderfully efficient! The average person could walk 35 miles for the calories in one pound of fat. Imagine if our cars could get such good mileage. Of course, when you're trying to burn a pound of fat, it becomes very depressing that you need to walk 35 miles to do it.

At any rate, fat is probably one of Mother Nature's greatest life-saving inventions, so we should try to appreciate our love handles for the brilliant engineering they represent.

It's no wonder that overeating is such a strong instinct within us. In fact, it probably saved the lives of many of your ancestors. The problem is that our current (very fortunate) situation never involves missing a meal. Yet, we still have the urge to overeat.

Fortunately, research is finding numerous ways to trick your body into wanting less food. Here are some relatively painless ways to reduce your appetite.

Sleep.

You're hungrier when you're sleep-deprived.

In my experience, sleep deprivation is the #1 way to insure a mutiny on your ship! If you aren't well-rested, you can expect to struggle with hunger, blood sugar instability, willpower and just feeling cranky, none of which help matters at all.

This one factor is so important for weight loss that you might consider doing whatever it takes to improve your sleep—buy a new bed, change shifts at work, create a Saturday night ritual of going to bed instead of partying—***whatever it takes!***

Even if you only manage a few good nights per week, it's worth it. It just makes everything weight-related feel easier.

Manage stress.

Chronic stress affects you much like sleep deprivation; it makes you hungrier, crankier, and weaker in the face of tempting treats.

Here's a test: Do you feel like you get away with dietary "murder" on vacations? Do you eat worse and exercise less than at home and not gain weight? I see this quite often in my clients and I believe it's because you're experiencing how forgiving your body can be when it's relaxed. It's likely a sign that your normal (non-vacation) stress level is hampering your weight loss efforts.

If this is your situation, try scheduling some weekly relaxation; like a bubble bath, hike, golf game or anything that relaxes you. I've seen stressed clients lose 10 pounds just from incorporating a weekly massage, with no other changes to their eating or exercise. What a painless way to see better weight loss results!

Slow down.

Take a deep breath, eat left-handed, set your fork down between bites or do whatever it takes to eat slower so that your brain has a chance to get the "full" signal.

Chances are, you're eating more than you need to in order to feel satisfied.

Get this: the average French person spends almost 3 hours per day eating and drinking. The average American spends less than 1 hour per day on these pleasant activities, yet is much heavier. No fair—how can that be? You guessed it: they eat so much slower than we do that they consume less food and fewer calories, even though they're spending so much more time tasting and enjoying food!

Avoid processed foods.

These are the foods that come from factories instead of nature. They taste great, but normally lack the unprocessed fiber, nutrients, protein, and water. These are all important for keeping your cravings in check.

Calorie-for-calorie, unprocessed nature foods always keep you feeling satisfied longer.

Instead of these processed foods:	Try these nature foods:
▪ Corn Flakes ▪ Bread ▪ Granola bar ▪ Protein bar ▪ Cookie ▪ Smoothie	▪ Oatmeal ▪ Brown Rice ▪ Fresh fruit with nuts or seeds ▪ 2 Low-fat string cheese ▪ 2 hard-boiled eggs ▪ Apple with peanut butter ▪ Nonfat yogurt with fresh fruit

Eat when you are (truly) hungry.

If you haven't already learned this from experience, let me save you the trouble. Going hungry never works in the long run because your appetite will come back with a vengeance. Your mild hunger that can feel so satisfying ("Hey! I must be losing weight!") will turn ravenous and make you eat many more calories (and later in the day) than if you had been eating reasonable snacks all day long.

This is one of the most common pitfalls I see. Whether you are consciously trying to stay hungry or just are too busy to eat enough, this habit will eventually backfire. Ongoing hunger will set off some alarm bells throughout your body. Remember that to your biology:

Hunger = Threat to Survival

This makes your appetite (and taste buds, metabolism, and brain chemistry) mutiny faster than you can say "Supersize it".

Plus, going hungry is one of the *least* pleasant ways to gain weight! If you're going to spoil your weight loss efforts, at least do it in one of the many tastier and more fun ways!

Drink plenty of water.

As people age, they sometimes lose the ability to detect thirst and experience this need as hunger instead. Drink water 10 minutes before eating to make sure you're hungry and not just thirsty.

Better yet, drink *cold* water. You'll learn why in the metabolism chapter.

Know your Avalanche Foods.

It's usually true that having "just a bite" won't do any harm, but *not* when it's an avalanche food. There are foods where, once you taste that first bite, you lose control and can't stop eating until you are disgusted with yourself (or the package is empty, or you feel ill, or you had the miraculous willpower to throw the rest in the garbage and pour dish soap over it so you can't go back!)

Don't feel bad if you have lots of avalanche foods—you're in good company. Even Benjamin Franklin wrote about having this problem!

Use the following worksheet to keep track of problem foods. Then, use all your discipline to avoid that first bite!

Avalanche Foods

Danger Ahead! The following are foods I won't buy or even *start* eating because once that snowball is rolling, there's *no telling* what could happen:

1. _____

2. _____

3. _____

4. _____

5. _____

6. _____

7. _____

8. _____

9. _____

10. _____

11. _____

12. _____

Avoid "excitotoxins".

MSG, Equal and Nutrasweet are in this category of substances that make food taste so amazingly wonderful and *unnaturally* pleasurable that you can't stop eating. MSG may be hard to spot because it can hide in food labels under terms like:

- calcium caseinate

- hydrolyzed vegetable protein

- autolyzed yeast

- hydrolyzed corn protein

- texturized vegetable protein

- yeast extract

Pay attention, and if these additives prevent you from getting satiated, add them to your list of "Avalanche Foods."

Eat a fiber-rich breakfast.

It fills you up and helps keep your blood sugar steadier for up to 18 hours. That means you'll have fewer cravings and less hunger.

Great choices are:

- veggie omelet

- oatmeal with berries

- fresh fruit with nonfat cottage cheese

- high-fiber cereal

Just make sure to drink plenty of water and increase your fiber intake slowly to prevent gas and discomfort.

Leverage your leptin.

Leptin is the hormone that makes you feel full. Calorie for calorie, some foods trigger it more than others. For example, cheese triggers less leptin per calorie than nuts, and fructose seems to reduce leptin output. Until researchers test other foods, pay attention and find which foods seem to trigger more satiety (per calorie) for you.

Don't forget to take the "per calorie" part into account.

People often say things like, "But that cup of walnuts was so much more satisfying than the cup of beans." That's because a cup of walnuts is 800 calories and a cup of beans is only 200. Find the better satiety bargain.

Embrace your food rut.

It turns out that a boring diet can actually be good for lowering your appetite! Research shows that people eat less when they eat the same meals week after week. Apparently your brain gets less excited about food so it's easier to stop eating.

Plus, it makes meal planning easier.

Look for excitement in *other* areas of your life besides food!

Pre-load.

This is the unappetizing term researchers use for a pre-meal snack. They've found that eating an apple, bowl of broth-based soup, or one ounce nuts 20-30 minutes before a meal makes you eat less overall.

Other healthy snacks would also work. Try low-fat string cheese, a low-fat yogurt, some snap peas, baby carrots, or any fresh fruit.

I suggest keeping some of these snacks in your car or office so you can eat them on your drive home from work.

Change density, not volume.

People lose weight more successfully when they concentrate their efforts toward eating the *same* volume of *lower calorie* foods. For example, switch your bagel into a turkey sandwich and you get to eat a larger quantity of food for fewer calories. Change your turkey sandwich into a turkey salad and you get even *more* food for your calories (assuming the dressing is on the side!).

One trick: Replace other foods with veggies. Because they are about 90% water, they are always very low in calories.

Bundle up.

Being cold increases your appetite. In one study, swimmers ate 30% more calories after being in cold water compared to warm water.

Whoa! 30% is huge! Make sure to avoid this silly appetite enhancer by leaving an extra jacket, hat, and mittens in your office, car, or school locker.

If you *do* find yourself chilled and hungry, make sure to feed the extra hunger with low-calorie choices like veggie soup, warm broth, hot tea, or an extra helping of steamed veggies.

Finally, pay attention...

...to anything else that seems to increase or decrease your appetite. If you find yourself stuffed, make sure to reflect on how and why you got that way. Then take action to prevent it from happening again!

In the meantime, here's your appetite-controlling to-do list:

- Make any schedule changes necessary to sleep more, even just a couple nights per week.

- Upgrade your bed, bedroom, sleep accessories.

- Schedule relaxing rituals on a weekly basis and treat them like the high priority that they are (i.e. don't cancel them!).

- Stock up on slow-digesting foods, high-fiber breakfast foods, and easy snack foods. Also, store away some soups, broths, and teas for a cold day.

- Put warm clothes in your car, office, or locker so you never get chilled unnecessarily.

Appetite Conclusions:

Don't waste energy trying to *resist* hunger. Use these tips to work smarter and prevent or minimize hunger in the first place.

CHAPTER 5:
Enjoy Your Exercise

Or at least hate it less.

If you're lucky enough to love exercising, then you can skip this chapter and we'll try not to hate you too much.

If you *don't* enjoy exercise, that's normal. To your body, recreational exercise is just a waste of valuable energy. Throughout most of history and evolution, it was important to save your energy for those activities that most promoted survival; like searching for food, building fires and shelter, defending yourself from predators, and evolution's favorite activity after eating, mating!

Most earlier humans spent their entire days exercising for survival: hunting, building, cleaning, foraging, etc.—so there was absolutely no need for

Mother Nature to create an instinct that would make us want to go work out at the end of the day. As mentioned previously, people used to walk an average of 12 miles per day carrying 25 pounds and still had to do many active chores on top of that. An instinct to *rest* when possible was the sensible gift Mother Nature gave us.

Unfortunately, this instinct to be physically lazy doesn't serve us so well anymore. Fortunately, research has uncovered a bunch of ways to make exercise more enjoyable and less painful; even if it will never be nearly as fun as eating or mating.

Eat more fiber.

It sounds odd, but one study found that people who eat more than 27g per day have better lung function. It's believed that either the fiber prevents inflammation or else carries antioxidants. Either way, the fiber is good for a bunch of other health issues too.

When your lungs feel good, exercise feels good; that is, until your muscles begin to burn, anyway.

Caffeinate strategically.

Caffeine makes exercise feel easier by boosting adrenaline, blocking pain, and helping you access fat. If you already drink coffee or tea, don't change your quantity, just time it strategically. Drink it about 30-45 minutes before you exercise and see what a great boost you get. You'll be able to go harder and longer with ease!

If you don't already drink caffeine, you could start with a little green tea, which has a bunch of great health benefits anyway. Green tea has about 1/3 the caffeine of coffee, so it's a safe way to start (unless you're on medications that don't allow it. Double check your meds to be certain).

Just make sure not to go overboard, as too much caffeine can give you the jitters or diarrhea. Sprinting to the bathroom is *not* a strategy for loving exercise.

Stay hydrated.

Studies show that being hydrated makes you exercise longer and harder for the same amount of effort.

This is one (but not the only!) reason that exercise feels harder the day after you've consumed alcohol, a strong diuretic.

The reason hydration boosts performance is very interesting; it increases your blood volume. You have more blood, so your body has an easier time getting oxygen and nutrients everywhere. During a workout, your body needs blood to go to your brain, your muscles, and to the surface of your skin so you can sweat and stay cool. Having more blood volume makes it easier to do all 3 at once. Neat, eh?

How do you know if you're hydrated? The best way is to look at your urine. It should be nearly clear.

Less pain, more gain.

Eat a carbohydrate + protein snack within 1 hour of finishing a killer workout to speed muscle recovery. You'll notice a big difference in how quickly your muscles bounce back. Good choices are:

- half a turkey sandwich

- nonfat yogurt

- eggs on toast

- low-fat string cheese and crackers

Don't bonk.

If your blood sugar gets too low during exercise, you'll feel like sitting on the ground and either sleeping, or crying. That's because your brain depends on blood sugar as its only fuel source (it can't burn fat, like your muscles!) and it ran out of gas.

Eat a few rice cakes or drink a little Gatorade and you'll feel fine again within a few minutes. Keep these "emergency foods" in your gym bag, especially when you're exercising hard and eating less.

Get enough sleep.

Not only does it make you feel better, but you'll produce Human Growth Hormones, which make your muscles recover faster. I like to think of a good night's sleep as the final piece of a hard workout. It's where your muscles do most of their healing and growing!

Avoid alcohol...

...for 24 hours before and after a hard workout. It can interfere with testosterone and slow down your metabolism. In essence, it makes exercise feel harder *and* cheats you out of some of the benefits of your workout.

If you *do* drink, just expect that first workout to feel terrible. Don't blame the workout, blame the Sangria!

Exercise-Enhancing To-Do List:

- Prepare your post-workout carb + protein snacks if you work out very intensely.

- Buy "emergency" Gatorade or rice cakes if you're in danger of bonking and put them in your gym bag.

- Buy a good water bottle (not plastic) to take with you during your workout.

- Make an appointment with a trainer if you need to learn a good workout routine.

Exercise Conclusions:

Don't be one of those miserable people at the gym who hate every minute. That's no way to live. Use these tips to train your body to enjoy exercise and to get more benefit from every minute working out.

CHAPTER 6:
Boost Your
Metabolism

When you burn more calories, you can eat more!

Fortunately for earlier humans, our bodies are great at adapting to new circumstances. One of these life-saving adaptations is the ability to lower metabolism when caloric intake drops. This allowed early humans to survive the tough times when food became scarce. It's safe to say that folks with unyieldingly *high* metabolisms were killed off during every winter, famine, or food shortage.

Interesting factoid:

There is a theory that people of Polynesian descent have low metabolisms because of how early Polynesians had to arrive there: via a very long boat ride. The theory states that people with high metabolisms couldn't survive on the meager rations that would be available on a boat ride so long. Only the people who could survive on a few mouthfuls of fish (or whatever else they could catch or bring along) made it to the island. They passed on their genes to generations of people who are lucky to be here, but who have such low metabolisms that they gain a pound by just *looking* at a piece of cake.

This same brilliant biology that helped us survive famines causes current dieters loads of consternation in the form of weight loss plateaus. This occurs when a person sticks to their great food and exercise regimen, but ceases to see good results because their metabolism conks out. The body thinks it's doing you a favor—the ultimate favor, saving your life during a famine—but really it's just frustrating you to the point where you want to scream.

Fortunately for us, research is finding plenty of healthy ways to outsmart your biology and boost your metabolism.

Choose unprocessed foods.

You burn more calories digesting unprocessed foods, like whole fruits, veggies, grains, beans, lentils, nuts, seeds, meats, or anything else that comes straight from nature and never visited a factory. This is because your body works harder to break them down. If a food was crushed, ground, blended, refined, etc. in a factory or a blender, the machinery already did all the work that your gut would otherwise have to do.

Save the work for your own digestive system and get a 15% boost to your metabolism. For an average person, that's 300 extra calories you burn, plus you're eating healthier food. What a bargain!

Lift weights like you mean it.

That means using heavy weights, lifting to failure, getting sore, and growing bigger, stronger muscles.

Every new pound of muscle burns an estimated 30-50 calories per day at rest. That's a lot of extra food over the course of a year (go ahead and add it up!).

So quit saying "I don't want to get bulky" and start saying "Strong is smart!" You don't have to bulk up everywhere; you can always add a few pounds of muscle to your chest, gluteals, and back where it won't even show.

I cannot emphasize this enough: If you like to eat, then resembling Twiggy isn't an option. You need muscle.

Besides, when you get older you'll be glad to have it. Anyone who fears muscle bulk must never have had a grandmother like mine, who was too weak to get off the toilet seat alone.

I'll spare you the details, but *embrace the bulk!*

Graze.

Your metabolism is higher for about one hour after you eat, and you also produce Human Growth Hormones with each snack or meal. Those are two great reasons to eat lots of small meals instead of a few big ones!

Just make sure to watch your daily calorie total. Frequent meals and snacks are great for your metabolism, but not if the calories add up too fast.

Finally, one caveat: if you're like me and find that *once you start eating it's very hard to stop*, then you may be better off just eating three square meals.

Drink green tea.

Research suggests that drinking 3 cups per day raises your metabolism by about 500 calories per week. Skip this one if you take blood thinning medication though, as it might interfere.

You can drink the tea warm or cold, regular, or decaf, although regular seems to boost your metabolism more. There isn't much caffeine in green tea (about 1/3 as much as coffee). It doesn't taste great but hey, 500 calories is worth it.

In addition, green tea helps prevent premature aging and lots of other health problems. This is perhaps the best "bang for your buck" habit in all of nutrition, so drink up!

Eat spicy foods.

They raise your metabolism and give you some well-deserved flavor now that you've probably cut back on salt, sugar, and fat!

Best choices for your metabolism are red cayenne pepper, peppermint, and ginger.

In addition to spicing up your favorite recipes, try adding spicy salsas to your eggs, salads, and chicken. Drink peppermint and ginger tea, and don't forget to eat the ginger that comes with your sushi!

Exercise early and intensely.

When you do a light workout, you don't burn many extra calories after the workout is finished. But when you do a hard-core, kick-butt workout, you get what is called a *metabolic afterburn*. Basically, you get to keep burning lots of extra calories for hours after you're done!

The harder and longer your workout, the more of a metabolic afterburn you'll get. It's not surprising that this means that longer, harder workouts get you the best results.

But wait! You don't have to sprint for hours because there's a time and effort-saving trick: *interval training.*

Interval training is the most efficient way to boost metabolism for hours. It's the workout method where you go hard for a few moments (anywhere from 8 seconds to 2 minutes) and then go easy until your heart rate recovers. You can do it walking, running, cycling, or on any cardio machine at the gym.

Just make sure to check with your doctor before you do intense workouts. A metabolism boost is great, but not worth risking a heart attack!

Avoid alcohol.

As a depressant, it lowers your metabolism.

Also, it's better to *eat* calories than to *drink* them, since digesting solid food raises your metabolism, but drinking doesn't.

"But what about red wine?" you're asking. "Don't I need it for my heart?"

No, you don't. There're plenty of weight-friendly ways to strengthen your heart, so do those instead. Walk, meditate, laugh, get more sleep, get a pet, volunteer, eat more veggies, take more vacations, whatever it takes.

Stop wine-ing!

Have good posture

Having a good posture engages the big muscles in your back and abdomen. It's been estimated that you can burn an extra 100 calories per day just by sitting up straight.

And as a bonus, good posture makes you look thinner!

Fidget.

Studies (involving motion sensors in underwear no less) show that people who fidget can burn as many as 800 extra calories per day.

This may or may not be for you, but let it be a reminder that even small amounts of activity can make a big difference over the course of a day.

I've got a client who does leg lifts when she's on phone conferences at work. Her employer may not love it, but it keeps her feeling great!

Drink cold water.

Warming it to body temperature can burn an estimated 60+ calories per day. Just make sure not to let yourself get chilled in the process, since being cold can increase your appetite.

Metabolism To-Do List

- Hire a personal trainer if you need to learn how to lift heavier weights properly.

- Buy green tea.

- Buy red cayenne pepper, ginger, and peppermint in the form of spices, sugar-free gum, or tea bags.

- Get rid of any tempting alcohol in your home.

Metabolism Conclusions:

These tips will help you burn more calories with minimal effort. It sure beats spending extra time on the treadmill, no matter how much you learn to love exercise!

CHAPTER 7:
Engineer Your Environment

"If you don't want to slip, don't put yourself in a slippery place."

Wisdom from Alcoholics Anonymous

OK, now that you're training your biology to help you out, it's time to fix the other half of the problem: your environment

As you well know by now, our fat-loving biology developed as an adaptation to the environment we inhabited. Our problem now is that our body adapts very slowly (over thousands or millions of years) and our environment has changed very drastically in only the last few hundred years.

In our old environment, food was relatively scarce, low-calorie, high-nutrient, not-so-tasty, lacking in variety, often rotten, spoiled or under-ripe, and a lot less convenient. That old environment also demanded a lot of exercise from us. In our new environment, there is delicious, clean, high-calorie convenient food almost everywhere and we don't need to move much to get it. If it weren't for our bulging waistlines and hardened arteries, we'd probably consider this one of humankind's greatest achievements.

Fun factoid:

Most animals become overweight when they are put in an environment with plenty of convenient, tasty food. America's fat pets aren't the only ones with weight problems anymore. Bears are gaining weight from rifling through campground dumpsters, and monkeys in Africa are reportedly getting fat on the leftovers of luxury game parks. The fact that dogs and goldfish can eat themselves to death suggests that nature never anticipated the problem of too much food, and that we animals are all the same, just following our natural instincts.

So the question becomes how can we change our environment to be a better influence? Do we need to move back to the wild to catch our own food and fend for our daily survival? Luckily no. It turns out that we don't need to take such drastic measures.

Research shows that eating and exercise are two behaviors that can be drastically influenced by relatively subtle changes to our environment, such as the number of people nearby, our dinnerware, music and even the weather. Often we are not aware of how these things affect us. Because some of these influences are barely noticeable, they make for wonderfully painless ways to improve our chances for weight loss success.

Again, there are lots of strategies, so choose a few that fit you best and give them a try.

First of all, make like a Boy Scout.

No, I'm not asking you to eat moss off of rocks, just that you *be prepared*.

Every strategy that follows requires some forethought and preparation, so accept this as an essential part of your weight loss plan. There's no way around it.

You can't control your food environment if you don't plan ahead. You need to foresee the food challenges you'll face and come up with appropriate solutions. Like the saying goes, "If you fail to plan, you plan to fail."

I suggest that as you fall asleep at night, think about where and what you'll be eating tomorrow. Figure out what snacks you need to bring, what groceries you need to buy, etc. If you can't or won't, then your planning could consist of deciding to...

Outsource it.

Pay someone else to buy groceries, chop veggies, or prepare your foods. If you don't control it, you can't flake, forget, or sabotage yourself. Why not make your kids earn their allowance by preparing you healthy snacks each day?

Fun factoid:

I was fascinated to learn that Oliver Sacks, arguably the world's foremost expert on behavior and psychology, outsources his food preparation. According to his interview on 60 Minutes, he's instructed his housekeeper to make the same healthy menu every week, and he keeps no extra food in the house. Perhaps he does this for reasons other than health or weight, but it's possible he's chosen to avoid relying on willpower to eat right, and this guy understands willpower better than anybody! Hmm, I take this as a strong endorsement for this strategy.

Carry a "Food Umbrella".

This is a snack you keep with you at all times for when the unexpected happens: you're delayed at work, stuck in a traffic jam, or your dinner host serves only fried lard balls. Good examples are in the list below.

Good Choice Food Umbrellas:

- low-fat string cheese

- apple

- hardboiled eggs

- nonfat yogurt (100 calories or less)

- Shredded Wheat cereal in a baggy

- bran crackers and water

- 1 ounce raw nuts or seeds

- baby carrots, celery sticks, or snap peas

- single serving of nonfat cottage cheese

- 3ounce bag of water-packed tuna or salmon

Don't forget napkins and plastic utensils when needed.

Leave emergency snacks

...in your car, office, purse or briefcase. Good choices are high-fiber crackers, a packet of tuna, or an ounce of nuts. See the Food Umbrella list above for more ideas.

I also like to leave an "emergency salad" in my refrigerator for those times when I get home tired, hungry and lazy. At those times it's extra important that the *easiest* thing to eat is also a healthy choice!

Pack up a backup.

Put an extra set of exercise clothes and shoes in your car, office, or anywhere that you might find yourself ready and willing to walk. Now you don't have any excuses if you forget your gym bag.

Avoid buffets.

Greater variety causes people to overeat. Plus, it's natural to want to eat more to justify the expense. One study found that people ate 30% more pasta when it came in a variety of shapes instead of just one shape. Yikes! And pasta variety isn't nearly as exciting as the variety in a nice buffet!

If you can't avoid the occasional buffet (I know they are ubiquitous for those spring holidays), ask the server if you can order a single item, like an omelet, instead of getting the all-you-can-eat option.

Serve fewer side dishes.

Again, since more variety causes more eating, you now have a reason to be a less ambitious cook! Go ahead and serve only one side dish with dinner, instead of trying to delight your family with lots of options. If they complain, blame me! Then tell them that if dinner is too boring for them, they are welcomed to jazz it up by performing skits, jokes, and dramatic tales of their day.

Avoid value-sizing.

Don't buy giant quantities of anything. It's called the "Costco Effect": The bigger the box of cereal, crackers or anything else, the more you tend to pour out at any given snack or meal. The bigger the cake, the bigger the slice you tend to cut. It's a lot like that principle in economics that shows people spend more money when they have more cash in their pockets.

You can fix this problem by using a measuring cup, but make sure to use it every time. Research shows that we all (even nutritionists) get sloppy over time and serve ourselves too much. In fact, the official (and depressing) statistic is that people eat 30% more calories than they think, because of "portion distortion." So don't get too overconfident in your spatial skills, no matter *how* well you scored on your IQ test!

Remember to count your 100-calorie snack packs.

Here's another great idea that backfired: snack packs!

Research shows that people actually eat more calories when they incorporate these innocent-looking foods. The theory is that these foods don't trigger any guilt, so we don't compensate for the extra junky calories like we would if we had eaten the same food from its normal guilt-inducing package.

It only takes 19 excess calories per day to add up to 20 pounds of fat per decade, so remember that *every single bite counts*; even free samples and bites you don't enjoy!

Out of reach, out of sight, out of mind.

Some great studies involving candy dishes prove that every little bit of convenience, proximity, and sight make a difference. People eat more candy when the dish is transparent (versus opaque), within arm's reach (versus just a few feet away) and in plain sight (versus hidden behind some folders). This suggests that even minor adjustments—like moving foods to a less convenient cabinet or to the rear of your cabinet—will make a difference.

Think of any tempting junk that is in your home, workplace, gym, or anywhere else. How can you make it slightly less convenient to get it? Again, remember that every little bit helps!

The closest gym is the best gym.

Don't join the nicest gym; join the most convenient one. Statistics show that most people quit going to their fitness club if it takes them more than 15 minutes out of their way to get there.

Don't multi-task.

Eating absentmindedly makes people eat more. This includes watching TV, reading, listening to the radio, or doing anything else instead of focusing on enjoying your meal.

If this feels too boring, then *good*! It's incentive to stop eating the moment you're satisfied and get on to your next activity!

Don't rock out.

Fast, loud music makes people eat faster and more. It's one reason that many restaurants use it— they want you to eat lots and get out quickly.

If you find yourself in a setting with loud, fast music, be extra aware of your eating and make sure to take a deep breath, chew slower, and set down your fork between bites.

When you're at home, experiment with different kinds of relaxing music. If your spouse thinks you're trying to be romantic, then all the better!

Drink from tall, skinny glasses

Unless it's water. There's an optical illusion that makes us think tall thin glasses contain more volume than short wide ones. People regularly underestimate how much they've had to drink when they use a short, wide drinking glass and they overestimate when using a tall, thin glass.

Get small black plates.

Studies show that people eat less on small black plates and more on large white ones. This happens for the same reason women look slimmer in solid black dresses. The color black makes a space seem smaller, so it appears as if the food is taking up more space. White has the opposite effect, making you feel like your meal is small compared to the plate.

This is low-hanging fruit. Even if you only take one less bite per meal, that adds up to tons of food at the end of the year. So put small black plates on your shopping list NOW!

Use smaller utensils.

You eat less when you take smaller bites. Ever tried to overeat with a shrimp fork?

If all else fails, use white lies.

If you can't get your friends, family, or waiters to help support your health and fitness goals, sometimes it's just easier to lie. Claiming a wheat allergy gets you out of eating baked goods; claiming a dairy intolerance gets you out of creamy sauces and cheeses. Inflammation of any kind (arthritis, say) gets you out of high-glycemic or processed foods.

Go ahead and lie when you need to. We won't think any less of you!

Environmental Engineering To-Do List

- Buy "food umbrellas" and "emergency snacks"— see the lists in this chapter.

- Put an extra set of gym clothes and shoes in your car or office.

- Buy tall, skinny glasses and small, dark-colored plates. If you don't already have them, buy small spoons and forks.

- Find someone to whom you can outsource your food prep—a housekeeper, child or the prepared section of Trader Joe's or Whole Foods.

- Put your "emergency snacks" in your car, office, purse, gym bag, locker, etc.

- Consider switching to a more convenient gym if you miss workouts due to lack of convenience.

- Get any tempting junk food as far out of your path as possible, even if all you can do is push it slightly out of view.

Environmental Engineering Conclusions:

Spending time and energy to optimize your environment saves you loads of willpower battles. Consider taking some time right now to get started!

Now let's work on your back-up plan for when your biology and/or your environment fail you. It's inevitable that you'll still have situations where Captain Willpower still has to save the day, so let's review ways to keep him strong and capable and there when you need him!

CHAPTER 8:
Strengthen Your Willpower

It only takes a 5-minute lapse in willpower to undo all your hard work for the day, so it pays to understand and improve this important tool!

No matter how well you "train" your instincts to cooperate with your weight loss goals, there will still be times that you need your willpower. You will have times when you're stressed, exhausted, caught unprepared and you'll be happy to have strong willpower as a back-up.

Many people feel guilty or ashamed when they have poor willpower around food, but I believe that using willpower to refrain from eating is *highly* unnatural to your body and brain. For millions of years, humans were rewarded (with the ultimate prize—survival) for eating as much as they could whenever possible.

Can you imagine many scenarios throughout evolution where it paid off not to eat the tasty, safe, and calorie-rich available food? Perhaps when saving some food for later or when choosing to give that food to a needy child or family member, but most of the time it was a folly to resist eating. Your brain's ancient wisdom knows that if you don't eat now, you might not get another chance for a while.

No wonder this is such a struggle for us. The act of avoiding good food conflicts with every basic natural instinct we have!

So don't feel guilty or surprised when your willpower isn't able to overpower your instincts. Use these strategies to understand willpower, strengthen it, and know when you can and can't depend on it!

Get to know Willpower...

On any given day, Willpower is like a battery, not a muscle. That means it gets run down with constant use.

There is only one reserve of willpower for all aspects of your life: getting yourself out of bed in the morning, being a courteous driver, being patient with people who frustrate you, making yourself study for that exam, etc. All these things deplete your willpower "battery" and make it harder to resist the next food temptation that comes around.

Most of my clients find that just knowing this one fact explains a lot!

It explains why teachers often lose willpower in September when they go back to school and have a load of additional demands placed on them. It explains why college students find it harder to resist pizza during final exams. It explains why it's so much harder to eat right at your husband's office party than at a party where you know and like the other guests.

And then don't depend on him.

Willpower is a fair-weather friend and he's undependable. Expect him to fail you frequently, and avoid relying on him whenever possible. As you'll soon see, there are many things that weaken it, such as stress, sleep deprivation, low blood sugar, distraction, and all kinds of things that might occur at any time.

So let me reemphasize: depending on good willpower to see you through a tough situation is like depending on good weather for your outdoor wedding. If you really care about having a successful event, have a back-up plan!

Conserve your willpower "battery life."

As I mentioned, willpower is like a battery and can get worn down from constant use. You can keep your battery well-charged by not wasting it on unnecessary temptations.

For example, stop meeting friends for coffee (where there are tempting pastries available), and start meeting them for walks, pedicures, or shopping. Don't put yourself in situations (like cafés) where just spending time there can drain you of your willpower. You might be able to sit at Starbucks for two hours without ordering a muffin, but that weakens your willpower for the next food challenge of the day. Conserve!

You might not think you have many situations that apply, but consider situations like this: A client, who was a high school teacher, used to feel so virtuous because she would resist all the donuts and goodies in the teacher's lounge all week long. She wouldn't eat a single one; hooray! But she broke down every Sunday and couldn't resist the free samples at Costco and the farmer's market, which added up to over 700 calories. As soon as she started avoiding the teacher's lounge, she had a much easier time resisting the free samples.

I see different versions of this story all the time. Research confirms that just *seeing* junk food makes you eventually eat more calories; somewhere, somehow. So do whatever it takes to minimize your exposure to temptations and reap the rewards of a stronger willpower battery!

Learn how to recharge your battery.

Just as frustration, effort, hassle and discipline can deplete your willpower, feeling pampered and indulged can recharge it. So here's some great news: it's not a foolish decadence, but a smart weight loss strategy to indulge yourself frequently.

Pamper yourself with inedible treats, like bubble baths, spa treatments, laughter, fun, and other relaxing activities. If you don't, your willpower battery will weaken until you take rewards where they are quick and convenient, in tasty, junky food!

I'm always amazed by how well this helps my clients. Often, when their willpower is bad and they are "cheating" more often, their instinct is to deny themselves any indulgences. They think "I don't deserve any fun or pampering, I'm eating like a pig!" But this is exactly when you *do* need to pamper yourself.

In fact, one lucky client even has a "Pampering Fund." Instead of birthday gifts, she asks her family to make a contribution to this fund so that she can shop, spa or otherwise indulge when she needs it most. Smart!

Manage stress.

In addition to all the other terrible things that stress does to your weight, it also weakens willpower.

If you know that stressful events are coming (e.g. a visit with relatives, holidays, exams, tax season) then *be proactive!* Plan some extra activities that will relieve the pressure, and make sure to do some extra "environmental engineering" in anticipation of weak willpower. For example, if the holidays stress you out, don't bake your all-time favorite holiday cookies. Instead, bake a recipe that doesn't appeal to you so much; or better yet, make a holiday stew.

Sleep well and enough.

Sleep deprivation weakens willpower. Again, if you know that a tempting situation is coming, make extra time for sleep and for the things that will help you sleep (e.g. extra time to read before bed).

Also, expect to be weaker on any day where you didn't sleep well. Try to avoid putting yourself in situations that require willpower.

I've got one great client who often doesn't sleep well because of hot flashes. If she has a big sleep deficit, she skips her family's Sunday pancake breakfast and sleeps in. Right on!

Use auto-pilot.

Focus on making permanent changes that can become automatic. Once a new habit is cemented in place, you can stop thinking about it. Research shows that habits come easier when you do the same behavior in the same way at the same time every day (e.g. eat an apple every day at 10am and go for a walk around the park every day at 4pm).

This is the best way to stop relying on willpower! Now think about some behaviors that you would like to put on auto-pilot. Figure out how you can make them happen consistently each day or week. Stick to it for that first difficult month or so and then Voila! No more willpower necessary.

You'll find no better investment of your time and effort!

Want more proof? Calculate the power of a habit. Just for an example, let's choose a really small one, like replacing one string cheese (80 calories) with a low-fat string cheese (60 calories). After one day, this habit will only save you 20 calories, but after a year it saves you 7,300, and after a decade it saves you 73,000. That's over 20 pounds of fat, or 80 sticks of butter off your body for that simple, little, relatively painless habit. Powerful, eh?

Think of other habits you could initiate—and stick to—right now.

Find commiserators.

And then laugh and complain about all your sacrifices and celebrate your victories. The social support will recharge your willpower battery.

I believe this is one reason why research finds that people are more successful when they tell more friends about their goals. I also believe it's the reason that one-on-one nutrition counseling has a higher success rate than programs that lack social support.

Don't be too proud to call a friend for support when you need it. Chances are that they will be thrilled to help you and glad to have you return the favor some time. Men, in my opinion, are notoriously bad at this. Give it a try and you'll be shocked by how quickly a good supportive conversation can make your willpower strong again.

Publicize your goals.

People are more likely to achieve goals when they make them public, probably because they risk embarrassment if they fail! At any rate, tell your friends and family about your eating and exercise goals so that you'll be less tempted to cheat.

Better yet, make a bet! Research also shows that people do better when there is money and/or competition involved.

Just remember to use your short-term competition as a springboard to permanent habits. It breaks my heart every time a local Weight Loss Challenge Winner celebrates with a gigantic pig-out. After spending 6 weeks eating like a saint—suffering to shrink their stomach, sensitize their taste buds, change their habits, and create wonderful weight-friendly biology—*they throw it all away* with the celebratory pig-out. Then they wonder why they can't maintain the weight loss. Devastating! (If you ever win a weight loss challenge, celebrate with something besides food!)

Forget moderation.

I know, I know, this goes against decades of nutrition advice. But, especially for those of us with addictive personalities, I stand by this:

It's often easier to give up something completely than to allow yourself small amounts infrequently.

Pick a few really bad foods (I suggest soda, Doritos- or Cheetos-type chips, anything fried and any sweets that aren't homemade) and just give them up permanently. It will be painful at first, but after a couple of weeks you'll forget about it. JUST DO IT. It's much easier in the long run.

It's a lot like training your dog to stay off the furniture: if you are consistent, your dog-like brain will soon stop whining and forget that it ever wanted to misbehave. If you let it misbehave once a month, it will spend the other 29 days pining for day 30.

Don't torture yourself like that. Give it up, get over it, and move on. My clients always hate the idea of this, until they do it. Then they love it.

Forget teaser foods.

If there are foods that never satisfy you; foods that make you just want more and more and more, then you need to give them up completely. You can't afford to waste your willpower pining away for the next time you can have a few bites. It's tough at first, but soon you'll forget about them and you'll have all that extra willpower to use on something else.

Keep a list of these foods so that you'll remember not to buy them or keep them in the house. Share the list with your housemates so that they can help you keep them away.

Ever been in a bad romantic relationship? Many of my clients mention that teaser foods are very similar. So be strong: dump 'em, get over 'em, and move on!

Food journal.

People always get better results and stay on track better when they keep an accurate and up-to-date food journal. Write down what you eat as soon as possible after eating. That means don't wait until nighttime and then try to recall the day's menu. And remember to write down *every single morsel*—you bite it, you write it!

Don't make food decisions when your brain is taxed.

The part of your brain responsible for good willpower is the neocortex, the more evolved region that also handles complex tasks such as decision-making, judgment, and trigonometry. When this part of the brain is busy working on a complex task (like memorizing a long number or figuring out solutions to life's sticky issues), it doesn't always have the extra bandwidth to make good food decisions.

If you know your brain will be preoccupied (e.g. during exams, while throwing a party, or during extra-busy times) then plan meals ahead of time while your willpower is still available to you. Also consider performing a junk food exorcism so that you won't have any extra temptations around.

Weigh daily.

It sounds obsessive, but research shows that folks who weigh themselves daily have more success. The theory is that you can catch yourself and make small corrections before you get too much momentum going in the wrong direction. Once you are too far gone, it's harder to get the motivation and enthusiasm back.

Play the "one good decision" game.

It's inevitable that you won't always have control over your eating environment. Surprises will happen, and there will be events where it would be too rude or awkward to bring your own snacks. When this happens, don't fret! Instead, play a game with yourself. Every time you eat, think of one good decision. Make it fun, creative, or kooky. Some examples are:

- Eat left-handed so you are forced to be slower.

- Drink a whole glass of water between glasses of wine.

- Excuse yourself for a bathroom break as soon as dessert is served.

You get the idea. One of the most important aspects of this game is motivational. It gets you focusing on what you *can* control, because there is always *something*. And every little bit counts.

I'm always pleasantly surprised by how well this game works for my clients. Almost everybody is able to lose weight during travel, parties, work retreats, vacations, etc. when they use this approach. Give it a try and let me know your good decisions!

Willpower To-Do List:

- Get a reliable home scale and use it daily.

- Start a food journal.

- Schedule a weekly activity that will relax and pamper you.

- Decide who are your supportive buddies that you can speak to when you need a boost. If you are doing my program, your Diet for Health Team should always be on this list.

- Publicize your health goals to anyone who will be supportive.

- Decide which foods just tease you without ever satisfying. Say goodbye, throw them out, mourn, and then *move on*!

Willpower Conclusions:

Like the saying goes, "The best defense is a good offense" and not relying on willpower is the best choice. But when all else fails and willpower is your only hope, these tips should help.

CHAPTER 9:
Avoid Common Pitfalls

These are the most common weight loss mistakes made by smart people.

There are a few common mistakes people make when they are working their very hardest to do the right thing. It always breaks my heart to tell them that their "shortcut" got them way off track, especially if they invested valuable willpower and energy doing something they believed was good. Don't let this be you. Read these common mistakes and avoid them!

Cheat days work great... For people who don't use them!

Boy, I sure wish I could change this fact.

Many weight loss programs allow weekly "cheat days" where you give your willpower a break and eat anything you like: No limits! No rules! No holding back! In my experience with thousands of clients (and myself), I've noticed that the people who experience great success with their cheat days always like the idea of them, but they don't actually eat very differently. Perhaps they eat a slice of pizza or an extra serving of bread, but they don't go overboard.

People who *do* go overboard (and why *wouldn't* you; after all, it's a *cheat* day! You're supposed to get to eat anything you want in any quantity!) end up gaining enough weight that they spend the entire week or more getting back to where they were.

Especially if you have a low metabolism, it's all too possible to overeat enough calories that you spend the next 7-20 days burning them off. Let's look at an example. If you burn 1500 calories per day and eat 1200, you'll run a deficit of 300 calories per day. A single morning Starbucks splurge (a fat-free muffin and frappucino) is 1500 calories. So even if you stick to your healthy eating the rest of the entire day, that one "cheat snack" has set you back 5 days!

Plus, a weekly binge prevents your taste buds from getting more sensitive and keeps your stomach stretched out. If you really need more flavor and junk in your diet, I find that it's better to add a tiny amount daily.

Of course, if the *promise* of a cheat day keeps you happy all week and then you don't really cheat, keep using it!

Don't confuse *nutritious* with *low-calorie*.

Nuts, seeds, avocados, olive oil (or any oil), coconut, pesto, hummus, dried fruit, and fruit juice are chock-full of great nutrients, but also calories. Every tablespoon of oil (no matter what kind) is 120 calories, which means you'd have to run 1-2 miles to burn it off! Every ounce of nuts is about 200 calories. These calories, while great for your heart, brain, and skin, still count toward your daily caloric intake. Don't make the mistake of thinking these foods are "free" just because they are awesomely nutritious.

My suggestion is to eat them, but pair them with low-cal veggies or fruits so that you can eat a reasonable quantity of food without overdoing the calories. For example:

Instead of:

- Peanut butter on bread
- Trail mix or Chex mix
- Guacamole
- Olive oil on bread
- Hummus on pita
- A juice smoothie
- Granola

Try:

- Peanut butter on celery
- Nuts, seeds + fresh fruit
- A few slices of avocado on a salad
- Spray olive oil on salad
- Hummus on sliced veggies
- Fresh fruit with yogurt
- Oats mixed with fresh fruit and toasted pumpkin seeds

You get the idea.

Remember, when you're losing weight, you have to think like a *calorie-poor person*. Just as a financially poor person needs to make every dollar stretch, you need to make every calorie stretch. Use them wisely. Eating these foods is like shopping at Sak's; you get quality items, but they are expensive! Be choosy and watch your quantities.

Also, don't assume something is low-calorie just because it's *wholesome, exotic, ethnic, vegan, from the farmer's market, or only-found-at-health-food-stores.* I once had a client who assured us for months that he was eating perfectly and not seeing results. He wouldn't keep a food journal because he insisted (no, *growled*) that he was eating *so* perfectly that a journal wasn't necessary. It turns out that he was eating vegan, which does *not* mean low-calorie. Unfortunately for him, he felt deprived and hungry eating all that vegan food, even though he was still overeating calories. Bummer!

Don't think protein is a "free food."

I think it must be the Atkins Diet that got people thinking this way. If you live in America and eat a remotely normal diet (even if you are a vegan) you're eating plenty of protein. You don't need protein shakes and you can't eat unlimited protein without expecting to gain weight.

It's true that protein is more filling, per calorie, than carbs and fat. But it's certainly not "free." Protein has 4 calories per gram, just like carbs, and excess calories from any source can turn to fat. Plus, eating too much protein can strain your kidneys.

Don't underestimate the importance of sleep.

Sleep helps with almost every aspect of weight loss; it helps reduce your appetite and cravings, improves your willpower, makes exercise more effective, improves your fat-burning body chemistry and brain chemistry. Sleeping basically makes the whole process easier.

If you're chronically sleep-deprived, you may have no idea how much easier weight loss could be. This one factor is so very important that I believe it is worth changing jobs, hiring a nanny (so you can nap), sleeping in a separate bedroom from your snoring spouse, or almost *whatever it takes* to sleep better.

Don't overestimate your exercise.

OK, this isn't going to be a very popular tip, but I see it so very often that I have to speak up. Many of you aren't exercising as hard as you think.

Now don't do anything crazy—get a doctor's clearance and all that—but if you're healthy and rarely get out of breath or get sore muscles, then you could probably increase the intensity.

Here's the bad news that many health authorities are too wimpy to tell you for fear that they will discourage you from doing anything at all:

- Walking is nice, but your per-mile calorie burn is only .62 X your weight, not a lot. And you need to walk more than 10,000 steps per day just to maintain your weight.

- Any muscle that you don't use (and you've got hundreds of them) is likely to be consumed along with fat as you lose weight: *Use it or lose it.* My personal rule is that I need to get at least one sore muscle per week.

- Any workout that you've been doing for more than a few months will lose effectiveness. Your body will adapt and cease to be challenged, making the calorie burn go down by about 30%. This means that as soon as your workout gets easier, it's time to incorporate something new and challenging.

- The National Weight Control Study (which tracks the habits of people who have lost over 30 pounds and kept it off) finds that it takes at least 40 minutes of exercise almost every single day.

- If you can carry on a conversation during your workout, you are probably not working out hard enough to lose weight and boost your metabolism.

- The calorie counter on your watch or exercise machine is counting the total calories you burn during your workout. What it's not telling you is that you would have burned a bunch of those calories by just sitting on the couch. Many people mistake the calorie count to be what they are burning *over and beyond* what they would have had they watched Oprah instead.

- Even if you have a personal trainer, you need to monitor your heart rate, muscle soreness, and perceived exertion to see if you're working hard enough. If you know too much about your trainer's love life, that's a bad sign. You should be working hard enough that you want to curse him, not have a conversation.

- Just because you're sweaty doesn't mean you got a great workout. Sweat indicates the warmth of your body and the humidity of the surrounding air. You will feel sweatier lying in a sauna than running the Antarctic Marathon. Use heart rate or perceived exertion as a better indicator.

OK, that's it for the tough love. I hope it helps. If you already push yourself hard, good work! If you don't, then get medical clearance from your doctor and see if you can start doing more. It will pay off in calorie burn, muscle gain, metabolism boost, *and* longevity.

Don't be fooled by health food impostors.

Food companies have an incentive to make you think their products are healthier than they really are. Read ingredient labels and be especially suspicious of shakes, granola, yogurt-covered snacks, calcium chews or "nutrition" bars, most of which should be called "candy bars with vitamins."

Unfortunately, even if the ingredient list and nutrition information looks good, you may still need to be wary. In fact, one study found that over 50% of bars and shakes were lying about their nutrition information. Yikes! So if they seem too good to be true; well you know the rest.

Always compare a snack to your "natural option" of fresh fruit, low-fat yogurt or string cheese, a salad, veggie soup, a turkey sandwich, etc. You'll usually find that you could eat a much bigger quantity of the natural food and it is more nutritious.

And please don't fall for the convenience excuse. You don't need a bar for convenience! Fresh fruit is nature's pre-packaged snack.

Don't avoid gaining muscle.

If you like to eat, you need muscle. Each pound of muscle, at rest, burns an estimated 30-50 calories per day. A pound of fat only burns 3.

If you add one pound of muscle to each arm, leg, and to your chest and back, you will not be huge or bulky, but you will burn 180-300 extra calories per day. That adds up to 18-30 pounds lost per year!

Muscle is also wonderfully healthy for helping you fight infections, preventing arthritis pain, and keeping you mobile as you age. So even if you don't care about metabolism, I say "embrace the muscle bulk!"

Watch the mind-mouth gap.

People eat 30% more calories on average than they think they do and they *burn* 30% fewer. This is depressing but proven time after time by research.

"Oh no, not me," you might be saying. But before you get too confident, keep in mind that studies find that even professional nutritionists make this error.

Measuring your foods and wearing calorie-monitors can help you be more accurate. Also, you can estimate your calories burned per mile of walking or jogging with the following equation: Calories burned=your weight in pounds X .62

Yes, I know that it's hard to believe sometimes just how little food your body needs to survive. It's depressing to us now, but it's the reason our genetics survived past famines and made it here today.

Heavy exercisers: don't be a morning hero and an evening hedonist.

This is the most common mistake I see among fitness buffs. They do a heavy workout in the morning and legitimately earn themselves some extra calories. But they don't *eat* the extra calories until nighttime.

I know what you are thinking. You don't want the extra calories after a morning workout. You're too busy, not hungry, and nighttime is when you will enjoy those extra well-deserved calories.

I feel the same way (and believe me, I've tried to get away with it), but here's why it doesn't work:

After a hard workout, your muscle cells become like calorie-sponges. They absorb extra carbohydrate and protein calories and then use them to make your muscles recover, making them stronger, bigger, and better while boosting your metabolism. You can eat extra calories and they will go into your muscles instead of turning to fat.: yippee!

Here's the bummer: your muscles only stay sponge-like for about an hour. After that they start to close up and your extra calories are more likely to turn into fat. That's why your "window of opportunity" lasts for only an hour after your hard workout.

Nature is cruel and suppresses your appetite after a hard workout. Like I said, I wish I could change this. If you're not hungry after your workout, try sipping on a shake or smoothie. In fact, low-fat chocolate milk beats out all other recovery drinks for heavy exercisers trying to burn fat and build muscle.

Enjoy your extra food during that hour and then be good come nighttime...or, if you *really* love to indulge at night, add an evening workout.

Don't overdo moderation.

This usually happens with my younger clients, so teenagers listen up!

It's true that you can eat pizza in moderation and ice cream in moderation and cookies, chips, fries, and cake in moderation, but when you eat them *all* in moderation, you are eating way too much junk food! If you take 15 different junky foods and eat each one only once a week, that's still too much daily junk food.

The depressing truth is that an average female can probably get away with eating about 200 calories worth of junk food daily, at the most. The average male can double that. When you look at labels and see how much junk that really buys you, it isn't much. Again, my advice is to think like a calorie-poor person and seek out the best calorie bargains. Popsicles, fudgesicles, creamsicles, and fruit dipped in chocolate are "good buys."

Avoid thinking "I blew it, so scr*w it."

In other words, never give up just because you can't be "good." Yes, it's true that eating poorly can set you back a few days. But eating *really* poorly can set you back a few weeks! So keep it together and fight your best fight! Even if you eat the entire box of Girl Scout cookies, but manage to throw out the last one (just to say you did it) that saves you 150 calories. If you made one decision that good every day for a year, it would lose you 15 pounds!

Every little tiny good decision matters. Never forget that. Every day you will be given different eating challenges and a different amount of willpower to deal with it. Always do the best you can with what you have to work with. Look for every opportunity to make a tiny good decision. I promise you'll be pleasantly surprised by how well this works.

Don't be social tofu.

Just as tofu will absorb any flavor it encounters, some folks will temporarily adopt the behaviors of their eating partners. For example, you may feel too self-conscious to ask for your dinner to be baked instead of fried or to ask for your salad dressing on the side. Or, you may figure that if everyone around you is eating a huge piece of cake, you deserve at least a half piece.

Wrong!

When it comes to eating, you can't assume it's OK to follow the crowd. With 2/3 of Americans overweight and gaining over 2 pounds per year, the majority is obviously not eating in a manner that is OK. So don't follow them.

If you feel like a bit of a weirdo drinking water while everyone else drinks wine, or asking the waiter for celery to eat with your salsa while everyone else eats chips, I applaud you. You're choosing not to be a lemming!

Plus, you'll probably inspire others who wish they looked and felt better too. If we don't start doing things differently, the whole nation will be obese and chronically ill. "Normal" for most of America is highly dysfunctional. So don't eat like them and never feel embarrassed for eating healthier.

Don't under eat just because you can.

I often see clients who are thrilled that they had a day (or week or month) when they were too busy to eat or weren't hungry, or were somehow able to refrain from eating for a long time. *This will backfire*, with your metabolism and probably with your appetite too.

In the short term it's thrilling because you lose weight quickly. In the long term it's depressing because you will gain the weight back without even indulging. This is the most depressing way to *not* get results! I say that if you're going to sabotage your weight loss efforts, at least have the fun of overeating tasty stuff!

Don't get leaner than you need to.

Every week I see many middle-aged clients who tell me that they used to be soooo skinny and now they can't believe how heavy they are. They don't eat junk or big portions and are understandably very frustrated. When we measure their metabolisms, we find that they burn so few calories that even eating a bare-minimum, near-starvation diet of 1200 calories, they gain weight. It's so very frustrating and depressing; yet I see it all the time.

I blame the culture of the 1960's-1980's, when women were encouraged to starve themselves to look like Twiggy. They felt beautiful then, but are paying the price now.

My point is *don't lose too much weight.* Weight loss can get addicting as you start to resemble a starlet, but it takes a toll on your metabolism. It's simple physics. Just like smaller cars use less fuel, your smaller, lighter body burns fewer calories than a bigger, heavier body.

Because of this, if you enjoy eating, I believe you should always aim to weigh the most that you can while still being healthy and feeling great. Yes, you heard me right: *be your heaviest healthy, happy self.* Find the heaviest weight that works for your self-esteem, blood pressure, joints, heart, etc. and work to maintain that. If you look and feel great at 150 pounds, why try to be 140 pounds? Sure, you may look slightly better naked, but that will require you to have a lower metabolism and to eat less; forever! For best chances of maintaining, find your highest "feel good" weight and stay there.

Don't think that maintaining is easier than losing.

Anything you *do* temporarily only gets you *results* temporarily. It's a common misconception that you can "diet" for 6 weeks and then maintain weight loss going back to your old habits. This is probably a big reason that 95% of people who lose weight gain it back again.

The depressing truth is that each weight has a set of habits that corresponds to it. If you don't keep the habits, you don't keep the weight.

This is why you should focus your energy on cementing lifelong habits. If you can once and for all, change your taste buds, appetite, metabolism, environment, routine, expectations, and habits, it will get you and *keep* you at your goal weight. Doing that is what this book is all about!

Conclusion

These are the best strategies I know for long-term weight loss success. They are smarter in the long run because they allow you to get to a point where you choose to eat right and exercise because you genuinely prefer it. They allow your willpower to be invested up front, to train your biological instincts to work for you, indefinitely. After the investment, willpower can work less hard, rather than fighting to make the right choice at every meal forevermore. In the long run, this is the much smarter way.

There are a lot of tips mentioned, and you probably can't incorporate all of them at once, so choose a few that seem right for you and try to turn then into habits. Once they become effortless, integrate a few more. And so on. I still continue to integrate more habits all the time, as I learn new ones or as the needs arise.

No good habit is too small to matter—even if the habit only burns (or prevents) 10 calories per day, it adds up to 10 pounds of fat after a decade...that's 40 sticks of butter removed from your body! With this approach, every tiny victory is an important part of your long-term success.

Finally, be prepared for set-backs, even with this wiser approach. If you're smart about it, every defeat can be an even *more* important part of your long-term success. Like they say:

Never regret. If it's good, it's wonderful. If it's bad, it's experience.

—Victoria Holt

Success is going from failure to failure without a loss of enthusiasm.

—Winston Churchill

When everything is going wrong, don't feel guilty. Getting off track is no reflection on your intelligence, ambition or character, so you don't deserve to feel guilty and it's not productive anyway. Chances are that your biology got the best of you. It will always win a battle here and there, but you can win the war if you work smart. You can always get back on track with these steps:

- **Wise up.** Reflect on what got you off track in the first place: Going too long without eating? Having a salty food with a sweet one? Lack of planning? Being in a tempting environment?

Make sure to get enough wisdom from your mistake to make it pay off in the long run.

- **Find a solution.** Figure out how to prevent it from happening again. Think outside the box. Be bold! One dear client brings her own diet Tonic water to bars and asks the bartender to put it in her cocktails without telling anyone. It saves her thousands of calories each year. No solution is too outrageous if it helps you to be healthy and happy.

- **Make your environment a good influence.** Perform a junk food exorcism and stock up on the right foods. Do whatever else you can to make your home and office your best helpers.

- **Get a good night's sleep.** If you read every chapter, you'll know why this makes *all* the difference in the world. Don't even *think* of skipping this step!

- **Start again,** wiser and determined not to make the same mistake again.

Good luck!

All my best,

Jill

About the Author

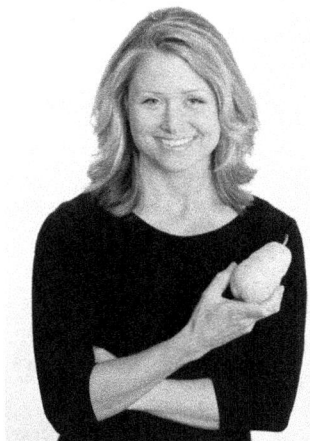

Jill Brook, M.A. is owner of Diet for Health, an award-winning nutrition practice in Southern California dedicated to helping people find their own most painless ways to look, feel and *be* their very best.

Jill received her degrees from Princeton University and UCLA and then worked as a nutrition and weight loss researcher at UCLA and the Pritikin Longevity Center, studying why *knowing* how to eat right doesn't help people *do* it. Jill now spends her time helping her clients work smarter at achieving their weight and fitness goals. She also writes books, leads workshops, consults for universities and food companies and occasionally appears on television. Visit her at www.dietforhealth.com.

www.ingramcontent.com/pod-product-compliance
Lightning Source LLC
Chambersburg PA
CBHW050536280326
41933CB00011B/1608